DEDICATION

To all my beautiful readers

Disclaimer

The information in this book is not to be used as medical advice and is not meant to treat or diagnose medical problems. The information presented should be used in combination with guidance from your physician.

Disclaimer and Terms of Use: Effort has been made to ensure that the information in this book is accurate and complete, however, the author and the publisher do not warrant the accuracy of the information, text and graphics contained within the book due to the rapidly changing nature of science, research, known and unknown facts and internet. The Author and the publisher do not hold any responsibility for errors, omissions or contrary interpretation of the subject matter herein. This book is presented solely for motivational and informational purposes only.

DRINK *smoothie!* HAVE A NICE DAY

Contents

RECIPES:

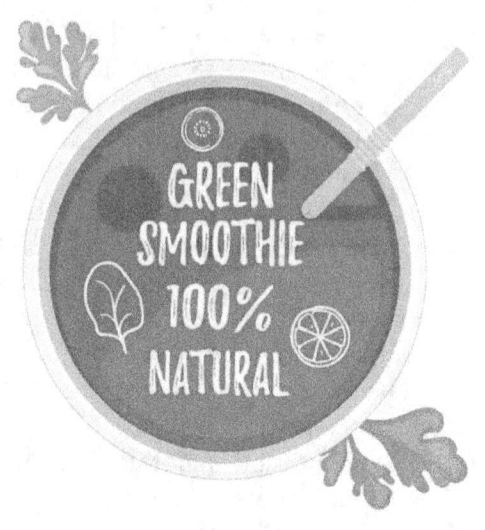

INTRODUCTION

GREEN SMOOTHIES

There are many different benefits of the green smoothies. They are like a true health bomb for your organism. Green smoothies keep your organism hydrated, give you power and energy, they are perfect for your digestion, skin and many other things.

Some of the green smoothies are kale, spinach, lettuce, collard greens and many others. The choice is actually not small at all. For those who are big fans of the green smoothies you can also mix them with parsley, watercress, and many others, the choice is yours. Really, anything that's green and veggie and you like it.

TOP 10 BENEFITS OF GREEN SMOOTHIES

By consuming these smoothies you'll enjoy many health benefits. Here, you will find some of them.

1. You can lose weight in a healthy and natural way

All people who consume green smoothies every day lose weight.

2. The entire day energy

Green Smoothies will fill you up with good energy. Drink it every day and you'll get plenty of vitamins, especially B vitamins, magnesium, minerals that will give you enough power throughout the day.

3. They are the healthiest

Surprised? Don't be. They are healthier then, watch it, fruit or vegetables juices.

4. Easy to make

They are so easy to make that if you are not a big fan of cooking and spending time in kitchen they will be your veggie favorite.

5. They are very cheap

We always think that healthy is expensive but not necessarily. They won't cost you more than a few bucks.

6. Picky kids

No problem. Mixed like juice green smoothies will look fun, taste well and problems with the kids and healthy food will go away.

7. Lasting energy

They are tremendous source of vitamins, minerals, fibers, etc. We are talking about the entire day energy.

8. Low in calories

They contain little calories but will fill you up for the entire day.

9. Glow

So full with the antioxidants, they will make your skin so shiny like never before.

10. Better sex life

Last but not least. All these great ingredients will improve your sex life. Try it.

ESSENTIAL TOOLS FOR GETTING STARTED

(Equipment - Blenders and Juicers)

In order to start living healthy life you'll need couple of things. Besides the ingredients you need the appropriate equipment to stir green smoothies. Blender or juicer, the choice is yours. Here you'll find pros and contras for both. Choose wisely.

Juicers are designed to separate the juice from the pulp, leaving you with a smooth, clear drink. Some of the juicers can also be used for other food preparation tasks such as mincing meat or grinding coffee beans. You can choose different look, size and of course different price. They are good for preparing all types of vegan drinks. They are good for making green smoothies but not usually good for different types of smoothies such as those with bananas and berries or nuts. And they've got at least 5 separate parts you need to clean.

Blenders are best friends of kitchen. The will provide you a good, healthy green smoothie in seconds. You can also use them for other things like sauces, soups and other similar things. The best advantage of blenders is that you get little waste.

Unlike fruit that is easy to blend for green smoothies you should have a blender strong enough to cut the fibers. You don't have to choose the most expensive, because the price is usually connected with the name. Fill free to choose the ones with the lower price and less famous name just make sure to check characteristics and strength. Once you choose the right equipment your healthy life can start.

We've already mentioned the benefits of green smoothies. There are many greens that will provide you the energy and supplements you need during the day.

Basil is a common aromatic herb. It belongs to the mint family. It is proven that it prevents a lot of health issues and that places him among most important herbs today. There are over 30 different species of basil. It is a great antioxidant, prevents diabetes, helps cancer patients, it is an immune booster, great anti-stress solution, etc.

Broccoli belongs to the vegetable family that also includes kale, cauliflower, Brussels sprouts, Bok Choy, collard greens, cabbage, etc. It has lots of nutrients but very little calories. If you want to start eating healthier broccoli should be on top of your list. Significant number of people, especially children is not a big fan of this green vegetable but there are a lot of recipes of how to prepare it to be delicious. Usage of broccoli decreases the risk of diabetes, cancer, heart diseases. It is also great antioxidant; it improves entire condition of your skin, body and health.

These things always sound good in theory but what about the taste. Well, green healthy smoothies can be very tasteful if you know how to prepare them. Well prepared, they will be good for any time throughout the day. Shake it, make it and bon appétit.

WHY GREEN SMOOTHIES?

There's nothing so healthy and good like green smoothies. Reasons for using them are so various that we could talk about it all day long.

They contain so many nutrients that they can actually replace your meal. If once your meal was full of fat or oil and you felt there is something seriously wrong with your body, you were gaining weight, you felt weak you should try this. It will be your breakfast, lunch or maybe even dinner but healthy and powerful. There are numerous recipes of how to prepare a tasteful green smoothie.

They are the healthiest and best smoothies of all. They can be so delicious that they could replace your dessert.

If you want to go on a diet use green smoothies. If you want to gain weight in a good, healthy weight-again green smoothies. You wanna beat up the disease- once more green smoothies.

Once you start using the green smoothies, for example in the morning, in the very beginning you will fill an extreme increase of power and energy. This can help you to overcome those rough days, full of stress at home, at work, at school, with children etc.

If you want to change your life style, start living a healthy life this is a true beginning. Most people think it's just a commercial, like something exaggeratedly written and talked about, but it's not. There's no person who started using green smoothies and didn't see changes. This time seriously, joking aside, ask yourself: "What good and healthy thing have you done for you today?".

WAR ON FRUCTOSE: DOES FRUIT MAKE YOU FAT?

Fruit - the first thing that crosses your mind when you here this word is most definitely "healthy". But, have you really thought about it? Are you so sure that everything related to the fruit is actually good for you? Well, you'll be disappointed when you hear that no, not everything about and from the fruit is good for your body. Sorry!

Generally, the fruit is good. We can't say it's completely bad. The thing is that it has to be consumed in a proper manner, combined well with other things you eat and drink or otherwise it can have an aftereffect.

It is worldwide known that the usage of sugar should be limited concerning even sugar from fruit - fructose. Some types of sugar like those from candies are not healthy at all. On the other hand we can't say that fruit isn't healthy. That's why things can be a bit confusing and it can be hard for us to understand the real danger of consuming too much sugar.

Fructose is a type of sugar found in fruit. Fruit is also a big source of carbohydrates. The level of fructose found in fruit is certainly lower than the one you can find in candies, sweeten juices and in similar stuffs, but if you exaggerate with these other things than fruit won't improve the situation especially if we talk about higher calorie fruit such as bananas. On the other hand fruit is full of nutrients, contains fibers and is rich in water. The only advice is to consume it wisely.

The problem of consuming sugar lays in the amount we are using. This amount has to be strictly limited. This is a sort of a modern problem since people have never had so many sweets before as we do today. Sugar is simply saying everywhere around us; in sweets, juices, sweeteners, etc. If you add any extra amount of sugar, even from fruit, there goes the trouble. It's simply unhealthy.

If we talk about sugar from fruit we should be aware of the fact that there are two main fractions: fructose and glucose. The enemy here is fructose. Glucose is the good sugar. It can be used as energy source and it's very important for some parts of our bodies.

There are many reasons for why fructose that we consume should be limited. It can only be metabolized by our liver and it's not an energy source. It harms the liver leading to the insulin resistance. It also promotes the growth of certain types of bacteria. We can talk about many other bad influencing facts of fructose but one is the most important; it gives the energy to the cells of cancer.

Since fruit has its good and bad sides; be careful. If you like it, consume it following these facts. Consume fruit with lower percentage of sugar and especially avoid consuming other types of sugar along with it.

SMOOTHIES AS MEAL REPLACEMENT OR JUST A SNACK?

Commonly asked question is whether a smoothie could replace our meal or not. We use the whole vegetable or fruit to prepare a smoothie. This is very good because this way we combine all important ingredients together. This food is full of fibers which can keep you full throughout longer period of time and it can also be combined with some other stuff such as butter (peanut) or avocado and other. Smoothies don't have to be green. They can be combined with some types of fruit. Because they provide your organism everything it needs, we can say that some sort of smoothies can replace a meal. They contain ingredients which are healthy, all the stuff you should have in one meal, give you enough energy, etc.

But if you prefer to have a different type of a meal and you don't want to use smoothies as a replacement for your meal it would be my friendly advice to at least add them to your daily menu. You could have them before breakfast or try making them your lunch.

So, the conclusion is next - it's not important whether you will use green smoothies as a meal or a snack, the most important thing is to introduce them into your diet.

If you choose to use it as a meal, the breakfast time is the best time to consume it. It will give you all the necessary ingredients that will provide you with enough energy and calories up until lunch time.

If you prefer different type of breakfast than these could save you from a fast food lunch which is, as we all know, the unhealthiest thing you can eat.

As far as dinner is concerned you may try to avoid drinking green smoothies for dinner. You can do this from time to time but if you are already changing something than breakfast or lunch are the best solutions.

SMOOTHIES VERSUS JUICES: WHICH IS BETTER?

This is still a big question since nutritionist can't agree about this one. In reality we'll find pros and contras for each. It will be up to you to decide which you will use, smoothies, juices or maybe both.

What are the advantages and disadvantages of them?

Well, generally speaking, smoothies are a mixture of the whole food and this is good because you keep all the nutrients from fruit or vegetables intact. Then, you can add some other high quality nutrients into this blending (this refers to yoghurt, healthy fat such as avocado, chia seeds, almond butter, etc.). This can be very helpful if you want to use the smoothies like a replacement for the meal. Your benefits from green smoothies are enormous with nutritional balance being one of the biggest.

As we all know, there is nothing perfect in this world. With smoothies it's all about mixing. If you use only one type of fruit or vegetables you can consume more servings than you actually need in one day. On the first sight you would say "OK, that's great. What's the problem?" Well, my dear, the problem is that this is wrong, too. There is a certain amount of each nutrient that is convenient to bring in into the organism daily. This is why you should be careful in order not to exaggerate. On the other hand if you take too much smoothies for dinner, although they are healthy, they might prevent weight lost (if you are on a diet).

If we talk about juices, they provide nutrients but leave the fiber behind. Fibers provide us some very important nutrients. When juices contain more fruit than vegetables they can pack much more carbs, more than you can expect. They contain vitamins, no one can dispute this but if you can it's better to use the whole foods, not only some parts because this will give the best results.

BUYING, STORING, CLEANING AND FREEZING

When it comes to buying green vegetables the most important fact is that they are not too expensive. This is how they are accessible to everyone who wants to lead a healthy life. You can find them fresh or frozen. They can be bought in supermarkets, at the markets, shops, etc. They are very available so you want have problems with it. If you want to buy a finished product make sure that the producer is checked, recommended by other people and most important that you are buying an organic product.

The best way to use green smoothies is to use them right after you prepare them, since this is not always possible here are a few tips of how to store them properly. Store your drink in a glass container with an airtight lid. Make sure to fill the container to the very top. This is important to prevent air from being trapped in the container as air will oxidize the nutrients in your smoothie (oxidizing degrades the nutrients in your smoothie, making it less nutritious.). Don't forget to seal the container tightly and store it in the fridge. An extra advice is to add some lemon juice to the green smoothie. The extra vitamin C will also help prevent oxidation. If you know in advance that you want have the time to prepare the smoothie later but you still wish to have it, make more and then store it in the fridge following the tips given above. Remember to by greenies of organic origin and to wash them before the usage.

Prepare larger amount of the smoothie and take some glass jars. Don't feel worried about putting glass into the freezer; everything will be all right as long as you follow the instructions. First, don't overfill them. There is even a marker on the jar that shows you the liquid limit if you are using them for freezing. After you prepare your smoothie, pour it in the jar watching out not to pour too much, tightly secure them and put them in the freezer. When you want to use it, take it out from the freezer and leave it overnight. It will possibly be frozen in the morning, but you can put it in a blender, add some water and mix it again.

CAN YOU LOSE WEIGHT BY USING GREEN SMOOTHIES?

Well, off course! Drink your green smoothie as a replacement for a meal every day. If you are really keen on losing weight you can follow this for four to six weeks period or however long you need to reach your weight loss goal. Try to avoid adding too much fat to your smoothies to keep the calorie count low. You should minimize the usage of, avocado, nuts, coconut oil, nut milks, almond butter, and tahini.

CAN YOU GAIN WEIGHT by using GREEN SMOOTHIES?

If you want to gain weight instead of losing it by drinking green smoothies you should increase the calorie content. Fats contain twice as many calories as protein or carbs. Choose fats that are cholesterol-free and high in nutrients. Combined with greenies these will help you put on some high-quality weight. You can also take an extra green smoothie about an hour before bed to help you gain weight faster. Have one green smoothie before or after your workout for a power boost recovery drink, and make an additional smoothie to drink before bed as a healthy calorie-loading snack.

DO YOU GET MORE PROTEIN, IRON, AND CALCIUM IN YOUR SMOOTHIES?

Green smoothies naturally consist of a lot of proteins, iron, and calcium. You can increase the protein, iron, and calcium content even more by using naturally high sources of each in smoothies you make. For proteins try focusing on, chia seeds, hemp seeds, sunflower seeds, almond butter, and tahini.

If you're interested in boosting the iron in your organism add cherries, molasses, dried apricots and off course more leafy greens (in powdered and whole-food forms).

If you need more calcium use homemade almond milk, beet greens, bok choy, turnip greens, collard greens, kale, and spinach. Make sure that all of these foods are of organic origin.

HOW ABOUT USING POWDERED GREENS INSTEAD OF FRESH ONES?

You need to know that fresh is always best. But sometimes you just can't get fresh greenies like when you're traveling or in winter, when some of them simply don't grow; powdered greens are an excellent second choice.

IS IT NECESSARY TO USE GREENS IN GREEN SMOOTHIES?

Well, the name says green smoothies. You can make a smoothie without greens all right, but then it won't be a green smoothie. The whole point of having a green smoothie is to get more leafy greens into your diet.

WHICH IS BETTER: A GREEN SMOOTHIE OR A GREEN JUICE?

The main difference between a smoothie and a juice is that green smoothies still have all fiber intact, while in juice they are lost. A green smoothie can be prepared in advance and also stored in the fridge for up to two days. But you need to consume fresh juice immediately.

ADDITIONAL DAILY VITAMIN IF YOU'RE DRINKING GREEN SMOOTHIES, YES OR NO?

It depends. Drinking a green smoothie provides a high boost of minerals and vitamins from real food with fiber. But you can't get everything from a green smoothie. Sometimes you may need to add something.

IS IT POSSIBLE TO OVERDRINK GREEN SMOOTHIES?

If you combine your green smoothies with a healthy diet, your body won't let you drink too much smoothies. When your body finally starts getting the nutrients it needs in a whole food form, you feel like you need more. In the beginning, you may want one to two liters a day. This is normal, don't be scared. Once your body is used to such a healthy diet everything will be arranged.

FEELING GAS AND BLOATING AFTER GREEN SMOOTHIE; WHY?

Drinking a blended smoothie full of raw fruits and greens after the diet full of cooked, fat rich, heavy foods this can be a shock to your organism. Your stomach may actually be low in digestive acids, or you may have an imbalance of god bacteria. The result is excess gas and bloating as your stomach tries to correct the situation.

DOES GREEN SMOOTHIES HELP YOU COPE WITH CELLULITE?

Green smoothies offer a powerful combination of fiber and minerals, and added hydration that allows your skin to detoxify, repair and rebuild. Weak collagen is the main cause of cellulite, as well as fat, and toxins. As you age, collagen production declines and causes weakening of the skin.

Dark leafy green vegetables contain powerful antioxidants. This will improve the production of collagen. Fresh fruits are high in antioxidants and vitamin C. So, yes, it will improve the situation. Try, you've got nothing to lose and yet you'll gain a lot.

CAN GREEN SMOOTHIES HELP YOU WITH WEIGHT LOSS?

This is one of the most commonly asked questions and the answer is yes, they can help (but remember-help) you deal with overweightness. First, you need to be aware that there is not a magic stick that will make your weight disappear overnight. This is a long time process (depending on the excess weight). No food or drink is guaranteed to produce weight loss; even if it's a green smoothie full of nutrients. To lose weight, you must lose more calories than you take in. Since most green smoothies are made from low-calorie whole foods, using them as a substitute for unhealthier foods you can lose weight.

The ideal recipe is to combine green smoothies as a meal replacement (one or two meals) with other healthy foods, avoid fats and other high-calorie but low-nutrient food and practice. Accomplishment won't drop behind.

INGREDIENTS TO AVOID

There are plenty of great foods and supplements to put in your smoothies that will give you flavor without excess calories. There are also some pitfalls. Too many people assume that any smoothie is a healthy option, but there are some ingredients that should be avoided if you are using smoothies as a weight loss tool. The most important thing you want to avoid in your smoothies is excess sugar. Even "healthier" sugar from natural sources such as fruit, honey, and maple syrup should be minimized. Canned fruits or vegetables: Fresh produce is always best, but when you can't find what you want, turn to frozen foods before cans. Canned fruits and vegetables often have added preservatives or sweeteners that increase the amount of calories. They have also lost a significant amount of their nutritional value. Fresh and frozen veggies and fruits maintain nutrient content much longer than canned products. Dairy: Dairy products like milk, ice cream, or frozen yogurt are common ingredients in smoothies, but they are chock full of extra calories. There are exceptions, such as raw milk and plain, full-fat Greek yogurt, which is high in protein and low in sugar, but most dairy should be avoided. Fruit juice: Juice is often high in sugar and calories and low in nutritional value, especially store-bought products. Many contain added sweeteners, and all have lost the fiber of the whole fruit. A limited amount of 100 percent juice is fine, but too much will just increase your total (bad) calorie intake. Protein powders: This may seem like a good way to get protein in your diet, but natural sources are a better choice when it comes to weight loss, IMO. Protein powders are good for bulking up and adding weight. For weight loss, stick with vegetables and other healthy sources of protein such as nuts, seeds, gelatin, and Greek yogurt. Caveat, for anyone that requires more calories than normal due to age and lifestyle factors, a reputable protein supplement is perfectly acceptable. Sweeteners: If your smoothie tastes very sweet, you are probably over doing it on the sweetener and potentially consuming too much sugar for a weight loss plan. Stevia is a natural, no-calories sweetener that you can use. Other good sweeteners, such as honey and maple syrup should be used in moderation. Too much sweet fruit: Whole, fresh fruits are good for you, and a natural way to add flavor and a little sweetness to your smoothie, but too much can be a problem. A lot of fruit in one smoothie can spike your blood sugar and cause digestive problems. A good rule of thumb is to stick to avocados and berries. Small amounts of sweeter fruits such as banana, apple, mango, and pineapple is fine, but keep those to a minimum. Smoothies high in sugar are a recipe for weight gain.

RECIPES

Sunflower Carrot Smoothie

Ingredients:

2 tbsp. sunflower butter or 1 oz. sunflower seeds soaked if desired

2 c water

2 medium carrots cut into pieces

2 celery stalks cut and frozen

2 cups baby spinach (or any green leafy veggie)

Directions:

1. Add the sunflower butter or seeds.
2. Add the liquid base.
3. Add the carrot and celery.
4. Add the baby spinach.
5. Blend at the highest speed for 30-45 seconds.

This smoothie has no cholesterol, and is high in manganese, magnesium phosphorus, potassium, vitamin A, vitamin B6, and vitamin C.

Grapes Green Smoothie

Ingredients:

1 c water

1/2 c red grapes

1 c chopped frozen banana

1 handful Italian parsley

2 c baby spinach

½ scoop protein powder

Instructions:

1. Add the liquid base in the blender first.

2. Add the banana.

3. Add the red grapes and Italian parsley.

4. Add the baby spinach.

5. Blend at the highest speed for 30-45 seconds.

This smoothie is low in saturated fat and sodium, high in dietary fiber, iron, manganese, magnesium, potassium, vitamin A, vitamin B6, and high vitamin C.

Superfood Goji Berry Green Smoothie

Ingredients:
2 c water
1 kiwi fruit
1 banana cut up and frozen
4 tbsp. goji berries
1 tbsp. cacao powder
1/2 c Italian parsley
1 ½ c baby spinach

Instructions:
1. Add the liquid base in the blender first.
2. Add the kiwi fruit, banana, goji berry, cacao powder.
3. Add the Italian parsley.
4. Add the baby spinach.
5. Blend at the highest speed for 30-45 seconds.

This green smoothie is low in saturated fat and sodium, and has no cholesterol. It is high in dietary fiber, vitamin A, and vitamin C.

Antioxidant Kale Green Smoothie

Ingredients:

2 c water

1 c banana frozen in chunks

1 c frozen or fresh blueberries

2 tbsp. orange zest

2 tbsp. orange juice

2 c kale

1/2 c spinach

Instructions:

1. Add the liquid base in the blender first.
2. Add the banana.
3. Add the blueberries, orange zest, and orange juice.
4. Add the baby kale and spinach.
5. Blend at the highest speed for 30-45 seconds.

This green smoothie has no cholesterol and is very low in sodium and saturated fat. It is high in dietary fiber, manganese, potassium, vitamin A, vitamin B6, and vitamin C.

Apples and Cinnamon Green Smoothie

Ingredients:

1 cup of water

1 c plain yogurt

1 apple sliced

1 teaspoon cinnamon

2 c baby spinach

Instructions:

1. Add the liquid base in the blender first.

2. Add the yogurt.

3. Add the apple and cinnamon.

4. Add the baby spinach.

5. Blend at the highest speed for 30-45 seconds.

This green smoothie is low in cholesterol, and is high in calcium, manganese, phosphorus, potassium, riboflavin, vitamin A, vitamin B6, and vitamin C.

Pineapple Cleanser Smoothie

Ingredients:
1 cup of pineapples, cut into cubes
1 part of peeled lemon
1 stalk of Celery
1/3 bundle of Parsley
½ of a Cucumber
1 piece of ginger, approximately 1 inch in length
2 cups of water (you can use coconut water if available)

Instructions:
Mix the ingredients into your juicer/blender. Blend for 20-30 seconds.

Your liver and your kidneys can greatly benefit if you drink this since the ingredients of this smoothie helps supports the processes of detoxification in these body parts.

Strawberry-Basil Green Smoothie

Ingredients:

1 peeled banana

6 medium sized strawberries

6 pieces of basil leaves

8 ounces of almond milk

2 cups of spinach

2 tablespoons of soaked (for 5 minutes) chia leaves

Instructions:

Put in the almond milk into the blender first before the other ingredients. Blend the mixture for 30 to 40 seconds until the mix becomes creamy.

If you have Vitamin deficiencies, then this smoothie is great for you. It is rich in Vitamins B1 to B6, as well as copper, potassium, phosphorous, Vitamin K and magnesium. It has 11 grams of fiber, which aids in proper digestion.

Super Detox Green Cleansing Smoothie

Ingredients:

1 piece of pear, small and cut into cubes

1 piece of banana, chopped

1 cup of romaine leaves, torn

1 cup of spinach leaves (you can also use kale leaves)

½ cup of chopped cucumbers

½ cup of chopped celery

½ piece of lemon, with the juice extracted

1 cup of water (you can also use coconut water if available)

1 tablespoon of mint, fresh

1 tablespoon of parsley, fresh

1 slice of peeled ginger, ¼ inch in size

½ tablespoon of chia seeds

Optional: 1 pinch of cinnamon, 1 pinch of cayenne and 1 pinch of turmeric

Instructions:

Mix all the ingredients in a blender until a smooth texture is achieved. Sweeten as necessary.

This smoothie recipe is a great recipe that you can try because of the benefits that ou can reap out of it. It has no cholesterol, low in sodium, high in potassium and high in Vitamin A, B6 and C. It is also high in dietary fiber and manganese.

The Super Green Smoothie

Ingredients:

1 ¼ cup of frozen mango, cut into cubes

1 ¼ cup of Lacinato kale leaves, chopped

¼ cup of parsley, chopped

¼ cup of mint, chopped

1 cup of fresh orange juice

2 stalks of fresh celery, chopped

Instructions:

Mix all of the ingredients in a blender and puree until the texture becomes smooth and creamy.

This smoothie recipe includes several ingredients that have diuretic properties that can help in eliminating toxins out of our bodies.

The Breakfast Blend

Ingredients:

2 cups of spinach

1 ½ cups of blueberries

¼ cup of superfood greens

2 cups of almond milk, unsweetened

1 piece of banana

1 teaspoon of spirulina Ice cubes

Instructions:

Blend all of the ingredients until it becomes creamy, frothy and smooth.

This smoothie recipe is a great replacement for a breakfast meal. It can help you feel energized and alert.

The Super Hemp

Ingredients:

½ piece of banana, sliced

2 cups of blueberries

1 cup of coconut almond milk

1 tablespoon of superfood greens

1 cup of spinach

1 tablespoon of spirulina

2 tablespoons of hemp protein powder

Instructions:

Blend all of these fruits and vegetables in a blender and add a teaspoon of hempseed oil if you necessary.

This smoothie blend is a great thing to enjoy at lunch. You can replace your unhealthy lunch meal with this and acquire essential nutrients and minerals without feeling guilty.

Alkalinity Bliss

Ingredients:

¼ piece of avocado, chopped

1 teaspoon of chia seeds

1 cup of spinach ½ piece of pear, chopped

1 scoop of hemp protein powder

¼ cup of coconut water

1 cup of almond milk Water

Instructions:

Put all of the ingredients into the blender and blend for 30 to 35 seconds.

This recipe features chia seeds which contains 2 grams of dietary fiber. If that alone already makes it a healthy substitute to sugar filled drinks, then tune out for more because it also comes with other fruits and vegetables that surely have healthy benefits for the body.

The Ultimate Green Smoothie Detox

Ingredients:

½ piece of peeled lime

1 piece of peeled orange

2 cups of chopped kale or dandelion greens

1 piece of medium sized banana, peeled and sliced

1 tablespoon of soaked (for 5 minutes) chia seeds

1 small piece of ginger, grated

8 ounces of water (you can also use homemade almond milk if available)

Instructions:

Except for the greens, blend all of the ingredients and push the "pulse" button for a couple of times. Set the blender on "high" and add the greens. Blend for 30 seconds or so.

This smoothie recipe is so great that it contains 9 grams of protein, 64 grams of carbohydrates, 321 calories and 25% of calcium. And oh, it also contains 4.2 grams of iron. Simply amazing!

Cilantro Detox Smoothie

Ingredients:

2 stalks of celery

1/3 bundle of fresh cilantro

½ cup of fresh pineapples, chopped into cubes

1 cup of green lettuce leaves

1 piece of ginger root, 1 inch in size

2 cups of coconut water

Instructions:

Blend all of the ingredients well in a blender. Puree until the texture becomes smooth.

This recipe will help eliminate heavy metals inside your body since one of its ingredients is cilantro. Since it also features the popular pineapple, it is also good for digestion.

Green And Clean Smoothie

Ingredients:

1 stalk of celery

2 sprigs of fresh mint

½ piece of avocado, sliced

¼ piece of cucumber, sliced

1 piece of kiwi

½ fistful of spinach

½ piece of pineapple

1 cup of purified water

A little hint of lemon juice

Instructions:

Simply blend all of the ingredients using a blender and wait for the texture of the mixture to turn smooth.

This smoothie recipe features everything green. You can benefit from all the fiber and nutrients, not to mention that mineral and the vitamins, which the ingredients of this delicious and healthy smoothies have.

Classic Green Juice

Ingredients:

1 small Granny Smith apple

¼ English cucumber or 1 small Israeli cucumber

1 small bunch of kale

1 handful green grapes

This juice is full of iron and vitamin K – just the thing for drinking before your menstrual cycle.

Vitamin Bomb Ingredients

Ingredients:

1 apple – any kind

1 fully ripe pear

1 handful of organic cherries (cherries can be pesticide heavy)

A pinch of cinnamon

This beautiful juice is sweet enough as it is but the cinnamon makes it something special for cooler days or evening.

Acne Healer

Ingredients:

1 cup kefir (coconut, water or milk kefir)

½ cup strong brewed nettle tea

1 Granny Smith apple

1 Tablespoon coconut oil

The juice of 1 lime

A big handful of fresh mint leaves

½ cup parsley – any kind, leaves and stems

This smoothie is a real does of TLC for inflamed and irritable skins. Nettle tea balances disrupted hormones and kefir and mint make sure that your system is cleansed from the inside out.

Spinach Explosion

Ingredients:

2 cups spinach, fresh (tightly packed)

2 cups water

1 cup mango

1 cup pineapple

2 bananas (regular sized)

Instructions:

Tightly pack your leafy greens into a 300ml measuring cup and toss into blender. Add water and blend together until all leafy chunks are gone. Next add in mango, pineapple and bananas and blend again; stop when all ingredients are homogeneously blended into a green liquid paste.

Use at least one frozen fruit to chill your smoothie.

If you aren't a big fan of bananas, feel free to substitute with another fruit such as putting in extra mangos. You can even freeze the bananas first to improve the texture of the drink and to also add some extra chill to your smoothie.

Banana and Strawberries Mix

Ingredients:

6-8 ounces of water

1 large banana

4-5 large strawberries, fresh or frozen (frozen preferred)

2 packed cups (or small handfuls) of fresh baby spinach

Instructions:

Once all your green smoothie ingredients are in the blender, put the lid on and blend on high speed until your smoothie is creamy and there are no chunks.

Carrots and Beet Jumbo Mix

Ingredients:

1 carrot, peeled, sliced

1 beet, peeled, sliced

½ cup red grapes

1 clementine, peeled

1 slice of ginger, peeled, about the size of a quarter

½ cup green tea

Instructions:

Steam carrot and beet until just tender, about 10-15 minutes, depending on how thick your slices are. Let the fruit slices cool to ambient temperature. Place all ingredients in blender and blend until smooth.

Coco Papaya Twister Thick Green Smoothie

Ingredients:

2 cups ice cubes

2 cups coconut water

6 tablespoon dried pitted dates

2 cups ripe papaya chunks

1 cup chopped kale leaves

Instructions:

Put coconut water & ice cube blend it for 1 minute. Now time to put papaya chunks and dried pitted dates It is time to put green now put kale leaves. Blend on high speed until a creamy and smooth puree is achieved. Now pure into glasses and serve. To improve taste – you can put almonds 4 table spoon almonds. Soak them first and remove the skin of almond to make them more digestible Garnish: Top of each glass place slice of dried pitted date, and papaya chunk.

This smoothie has kale it is low in calorie, high in fiber and has zero fat. Kale is rich source of iron, Vitamin, and kale is powerful antioxidants it will also help you with cardiovascular support and Vitamin A not only you are drinking a tasty smoothie but in fact this will help you to detoxify your body.

Avocado Buster Limes

Ingredients:

6 piece ice cubes

1 cup Unsweetened coconut water

½ avocado fruit

2 whole limes

1 sliced apple

1tablespoon honey

Instructions:

Pluck out the leaves of the spinach. Discard stems. Remove seed of avocado. Using a spoon, scoop out flesh the peeling. Peal and quarter limes. Cut apple into half –inch slices. In a blender, place apple, avocado, spinach and lime. Add ice cubes and 1 tablespoon honey and coconut water. Blend all ingredients until smooth. Pour into glass and drink fresh.

Garnish: Top of each glass place thin apple slice.

Avocado is a green part of this smoothie It will help you with antioxidant carotenoids, vitamin e and vitamin c it is also helpful for skin care also and this smoothies help you with diabetes and arthritis. More of a juice than a smoothie (because of the ingredient's low fiber content), this invigorating frappe alkalizes and hydrates the body. That is why this drink is perfect for right after a strenuous workout or when it's hot outside. In fact, I highly recommend you add this to the menu for all of your midsummer picnics and sporting events. It's tasty, light, and refreshing.

Broccoli Apple Combo Smoothie

Ingredients:
½ cup broccoli heads
1 cup spinach
1 green apple
1 orange
1 cup Coconut milk
½ cup chopped cantaloupe
1 cup ice cubes

Instructions:
Wash the spinach under running water. Peel orange. Separate into segments. Peel and core apple. Cut them into ½ inch cubes. Put all ingredients into blender and blend it for 4 minutes at high speed until it all mix up well. Pour into glass and serve it.

Cantaloupe is the most popular variety of melon in the United States and it's easy to see why. Succulently sweet and a great source of beta-carotene, a powerful antioxidant, this fruit is nothing less than a big ball of joy. Here I've dressed it up with a handful of herbs and a touch of extra sweetness. Fresh spinach leaves are rich source of several vital anti-oxidant vitamins like vitamin A, vitamin C, and flavonoid poly phenolic antioxidants such as lutein, zea-xanthin and beta also spinach will help you with your weight reduction.

Cool Kale Mint Smoothie

Ingredients:

Cup chopped kale leaves

15 pieces mint leaves

4 whole pitted dates

2 tablespoon raw cashew

1 ½ cup coconut milk

Instructions:

Put all ingredients in a blender. Whiz on high speed until smooth. Pour into glasses and serve immediately. Make it better - If you like to change the taste try to put 1 cup ice cube for cold treat.

Kale is such a delicate and beautiful little green. Kale is a very versatile and nutritious green leafy vegetable. It is a widely popular vegetable since ancient Greek and Roman times for its low fat, no cholesterol but health benefiting anti-oxidant properties. It adds a peppery flavor to this smooth drink that is very reminiscent of horseradish. I love everything about this smoothie and with the little kale leaves for garnish, it's as gorgeous as it is tasty.

Tangy Minty Green Smoothie

Ingredient:

10 leaves coriander

10 leaves of mint

10 leaves of sweet basil

2 Ripe orange

½ small avocado fruit

½ cup cucumber slices

Juice of ½ lime fruit

½ cup distilled water

Instructions:

Peel orange and separate them, remove seeds. Scoop the flesh from the avocado fruit. Slice cucumber in to half-inch thickness. Put all ingredients in a blender in this order mint, basil, coriander, orange, avocado, cucumber, lime juice. Blend on high speed until smooth. Pour into glass and serve fresh.

Our modern day lives expose us to a myriad of toxins. Whether it is car exhaust or pesticides, it all adds to our toxic load. Beets are thought to have the amazing ability to cleanse poisons like these from the body. This simple frappe will refresh you, while alkalizing and purifying your body of the toxins we accumulate on a daily basis. Green part of this smoothie is avocado which will help you with your weight loss and skin benefit.

BB Magic Smoothie

Ingredients:

1 cup broccoli

2 cups diced ripe bananas

½ cup distilled water

½ cup ice cubes

Instructions:

Rinse broccoli in running water and clean thoroughly. Peel bananas and cut into 1-inch slices. Put all ingredients in a blender and whiz until smooth. Pour into a glass and enjoy.

Your mom always told you to eat your broccoli and this smoothie will definitely do the trick. It's just like the famous juice, but with the added benefit of fiber. And with so many vitamins and minerals, it's like a multivitamin in a glass. Smart and delicious, with every sip of this smoothie, you make your mother proud!

Cocaberry Super Detox Smoothie

Ingredients:

2 cups romaine lettuce

1 ½ cups fresh blackberry

3 piece pitted date (pre- soaked)

½ cup almond milk

½ cup coconut milk

½ cup ice cubes

Instructions:

Blend romaine lettuce, milk and water until smooth. Add in the rest of ingredients and continue blending until thoroughly mixed. Pour into tall glasses and serve immediately.

Can you say super fruit? Blackberries are a powerhouse of health-boosting nutrients like phytochemicals and antioxidants, which may help fight cancer. But that's not even why I recommend this smoothie for weight loss. This is the smoothie to grab when you are craving something sweet, but don't want to go overboard. It helps you get your sugar fix without cheating.

Green Spinach Peaches Twist Smoothie

Ingredients:

½ cup spinach

½ cup Brussels sprouts

2 medium peaches

2 medium banana

½ cup green tea

1 cup Fresh raspberries

Instructions:

Rinse spinach & Brussels sprouts in running water and clean thoroughly. Remove seed from peaches with the tablespoon. First put green in the blender with green tea whiz until smooth Now time to put rest of the ingredient into blender and blend until smooth. Pour it in the glass and drink fresh.

This frappe is one of my all-time favorite drinks. If you are a green tea lover, you will go nuts for it. The grassy flavor of the spinach accentuates the tea perfectly and grapes add a subtle sweetness. The antioxidants, vitamins, and minerals in this tasty concoction are just icing on the cake. Spinach is store house for many phyto-nutrients that have health promotional and disease prevention properties.

Simple But Strong Berries Lettuce Smoothie

Ingredients:
1 cup chopped romaine lettuce
2 cups fresh blackberries
½ tablespoon lemon zest
1 large banana
5 mint leaves
1 cup ice cubes
½ cup chopped zucchini

Instructions:
First put chopped romaine lettuce & and zucchini in blender and whiz until smooth. Now peel and cut in to slice banana. Put all ingredients in the blender, and blend them until smooth Pour it into a glass and drink fresh.

Forget the cocktail! Renew yourself after a long day with this delicious smoothie. Relax knowing that you will be bolstering up your immune system with vitamin C and tons of antioxidants. Better yet, invite friends over and share this mock-tail with them. They'll be shocked and delighted when they learn that they just drank a boat load of healthy vegetables! Romaine lettuce Fresh leaves contain good amounts folates and vitamin C. Folates are part of co-factors in the enzyme metabolism required for DNA synthesis and therefore, play a vital role in prevention of the neural tube defects in the baby (fetus) during pregnancy.

Rich Mango - Broccoli Milk Smoothie

Ingredients:

1 cup almond milk

½ cup coconut milk

1 whole medium sized ripe mango

½ cup frozen banana

4 medium sized broccoli heads

1 cup ice cubes

Instructions:

Wash and prepare all ingredients. Peel the mango, remove the seed and slice onto 2- inch cubes. Juice the lime fruit. Pour coconut milk into blender & almond milk add mango, banana and lime juice. Add broccoli last. Blend all ingredients on high speed until smoothie reaches a creamy consistency (This will take about 30 seconds to process). Pour into a glass and serve fresh.

Ready to indulge? This smoothie feels like dessert while filling you and your family up for the long day ahead. And the best part, it tastes just like pie! This recipe is perfect for kids, too. They'd never guess that they are fueling up on fiber, beta-carotene, healthy fats, and antioxidants. It's a treat for your taste buds as well as your health. This smoothie is very low in calorie it is rich in dietary fiber, minerals, vitamins, and anti-oxidants that have proven health benefits.

3 Fruit One Green Thick Smoothie

Ingredient:

½ cup Brussels sprouts

½ cup ripe mango chunks

½ cup diced ripe bananas

½ cup muesli

½ cup pineapple

1 tablespoon sesame seeds

¼ cup pitted dates

½ cup non-dairy milk

½ cup ice cubes

Instructions:

Place water, milk, muesli and I Brussels sprouts in a blender. Mix thoroughly. Add remaining ingredients and continue blending until smooth Pour into glass and drink fresh.

Break out the beach chairs and sun hats; it's time for a trip to the beach! While you and your family may not have the opportunity to step out of your house today, but this smoothie will make you feel like you are in the Bahamas. It features a mouthwatering combination of luscious tropical fruits. They are packed with antioxidants, and the best part, they are absolutely delicious!

Dairy Berry Green Smoothie

Ingredients:

½ cup spinach

½ cup sliced bananas

½ cup blueberries

½ cup non- dairy milk

½ cup oats

1 tablespoon sunflower seeds

½ cup ice cubes

½ cup water

Instructions:

Put ice cubes, water, spinach and oats in a blender. Blend on high speed until mixed. Add milk blueberries, bananas and sunflower seeds. Blend until smooth. Pour into a tall glass and serve.

Ready for something a little outside the box? This mouthwatering smoothie is a combination of tart blueberries, sweet banana, and an effervescent twist. Sunflower seeds just a little something that will leave you thinking and wanting more! Try sharing this daring drink and see if your friends and family can guess the secret ingredient.

Grape Celery Power Smoothie

Ingredients:

1 cup black grapes.

1 large stalk of celery

½ cup instant oats

1 tablespoon pumpkin seeds

½ cup oat milk

½ cup coconut water

½ cup ice cubes

Instructions:

Cut celery into 2-inch strips so it becomes easier to process. Put celery, oats, ice cubes and water in a blender and whiz on high speed until smooth. Add black grapes, pumpkin seed and milk blend until smooth. Pour into a glass and drink fresh.

Believe it or not, coconut water has been administered to dehydrated patients via IV straight into their veins. This is because it is perfectly balanced to restore the body's fluids and is full of electrolytes. After a long day at work or a good workout, it's not uncommon to feel dehydrated. This soothing smoothie is the perfect way to replenish your body's water balance while indulging in a delicious treat. This smoothie also helps you with your joint pains, lung infections and asthma.

Vanilla Coconut Green Smoothie

Ingredients:

1 cup kale leaves

½ cup Oats

½ teaspoon vanilla extract

A pinch of salt

¼ cup unsweetened coconut milk

½ cup ice cubes

Instructions:

Blend kale leaves and water first. When smooth, add oats, Vanilla extract, salt, coconut milk and ice cubes and blend until fully mixed. Pour into a glass and serve.

When you think of a powerhouse of nutrition, dark leafy greens always come to mind. They are a great source of vitamins like B, K, C, and E along with many essential minerals. This smoothie is a great one for those of you who are trying to become more accustomed to the flavor of greens. That's because I paired them up with tangy green and sweet vanilla for a smoothie that is green, but with a hint of sweetness.

Lemon Forest Green Smoothie

Ingredients:

½ cup pineapple

¼ cup cauliflower florets

½ cup pink grapefruit

½ tablespoon linseeds

1 tablespoon lemon zest

½ tablespoon almond nuts

2 tablespoon dried pitted dates (pre-soaked for a smoother blend)

1/4 cup dried apricots

½ cup non- dairy milk

Instructions:

Put water, milk, broccoli, Pineapple, cauliflower and grapefruit in a blender. Whiz until, mixed thoroughly. Add linseeds, almonds, dates and apricots. Blend until smooth. Pour into a tall glass and enjoy.

Dreamy and creamy, this smoothie is like a melted Popsicle in a cup. And even though it's green, you'd never guess by its bright and fresh flavor that cauliflower florets have worked its way into the mix. Don't let the sweet, light flavor fool you either. This smoothie is packed with iron, protein, and fiber which make for a substantial drink.

Yogurt Peach Green Smoothie

Ingredients:

1 cup romaine lettuce

3 small whole peaches

1 tablespoon sesame seeds

¼ cup dried apricots(pre-soaked for a smoother blend)

½ cup non – dairy milk

½ cup non-dairy yogurt

½ cup ice cubes

Instructions:

Blend in romaine lettuce, milk and yogurt until smooth. Add all remaining ingredients and process in the blender until thoroughly, mixed. Pour into a glass and drink immediately.

For me, the heavy green flavor of dark leafy vegetables has been an acquired taste. That doesn't apply to this smoothie. Because of the addition of fresh flavors like dill, romaine lettuce, and citrus this smoothie is light and refreshing. It's a tasty combination that, if you are not a greens person, you will be glad you tried.

Green Hurricane Delta Detox Smoothie

Ingredients:

½ cup spinach

½ kale leaves

¼ romaine lettuce

4 broccoli heads

Medium stalk of celery

¼ cup parsley leaves

¼ cup Brussels sprouts

5 mint leaves

3 medium lemon

Pinch of sea salt

1 cup ice cubes

Instructions:

First peel lemon and square them. Put rest of the ingredient in the blender. Whiz until smooth Pour into glass and drink fresh.

This smoothie is dedicated to all of the die-hard green smoothie addicts out there. This is the most hard core leafy green smoothie in this book. Please don't let that scare you off, though. The fresh lime lightens up the flavor quite a bit. There's even a bit of neutral zucchini thrown in the mix for a balanced, yet unmistakably green, drink.

Gleaming Green Spinach and Lettuce Smoothie

Ingredients:

3 cups chopped romaine lettuce (or about 1 head)
2 cups chopped spinach leaves (about half of a large bunch)
½ cup sliced celery
½ cup diced apples (about ½ medium sized whole)
¼ cup diced pear (about 1 medium sized wholes)
½ cup sliced banana
½ tablespoon fresh lemon juice
1 cup water

Instructions:

Wash all vegetables and fruits thoroughly before handling them. Put romaine lettuce, spinach and water together in a blender. Process at low speed until mixture becomes smooth. Add celery, apple and pear. Blend mixture at high speed. Lastly, add the banana and lemon juice and puree until well blended. Pour into glasses and serve fresh.

Variation:

Add ½ cup each of parsley and cilantro for an even greener smoothie. Using stems are okay, but chop them so they do not ruin your blender or smoothie maker. Add an inch of ginger to recipe for an extra zing.

This smoothie is 7 parts green vegetables and 3 parts fruit, so this will help you put more greens into your diet than you normally could in one sitting. This well-mixed green smoothie is easy to digest, which will make your body absorb more vitamins and minerals. Plus, this smoothie is amazingly filling, so it will keep you from reaching for that carbohydrate packed snack just to pacify your hunger pangs.

Energy Booster Spinach and Collard Greens Smoothie

Ingredients:

1 cup fresh spinach

1 cup fresh collard greens

4 whole medium sized oranges

3 cups pineapple chunks

Instructions:

Squeeze out the juice from the oranges. Use this fresh juice as liquid base for blending the spinach and collard greens together. Blend at slow speed until smooth. Add the pineapples to the orange and greens mixture and blend at high speed until well mixed. Pour and serve immediately.

Variation: Want this smoothie to double as a cold thirst quencher? Add 6 ice cubes into the mix and blend until smooth. Can't find collard greens? Take it easy by replacing with a cup of chopped kale.

Packed with fruits and vegetables that are rich in minerals, proteins and vitamins A, C, E and K, this smoothie is a surefire energy booster that will allow your body to function at an optimal level. That's real, green and mean energy in a glass!

Green Piña Colada Smoothie

Ingredients:
1 cup chopped dandelion greens
4 cups fresh ripe pineapple chunks
½ cup shredded coconut meat
4 tablespoons dried pitted dates
2 cups unsweetened coconut water
2 cups ice cubes

Instructions:
Put all ingredients in a blender. Remember to put the liquid first and the greens last. Add ingredients in between. Blend on high speed until a creamy and smooth puree is achieved. Pour into glasses and serve.

Variation: For a nutty taste, add 4 tablespoons raw cashew nuts to the recipe. Just be sure to choose the right cashews (plump, uniform in color, smells nutty and sweet) and always soak them first to remove enzyme inhibitors and make them more digestible.

Dandelion greens may be bitter when eaten raw, but adding this super green vegetable to the mix will make your smoothie taste like it has alcohol in it. Best of all, dandelion greens are said to be the ultimate detox and cleansing green because it is a great liver cleanser.

Kiwi Green Smoothie

Ingredients:

1 cup chopped kale leaves

1 cup chopped Romaine lettuce

1 cup chopped Swiss chard leaves

½ cup sliced ripe bananas

½ kiwi fruit juice of ½ lemon

1 cup distilled water

1 teaspoon bee pollen

½ teaspoon maca powder

Instructions:

Wash all ingredients thoroughly. Prepare as directed in the recipe. Put all ingredients in a blender. Blend at high speed until smooth. Pour into a glass and serve immediately.

Variation: Replace water with same amount of unsweetened coconut water for extra alkaline in your green smoothie. If kiwis are not in season, substitute it with mango or papaya.

Adding nutrition supplements like bee pollen and maca powder in your green smoothie will increase health benefits that your body will acquire from your mix.

Minty Green Smoothie

Ingredients:

1 cup chopped spinach leaves

10 pieces mint leaves

2 whole pitted dates

2 tablespoons raw cashew butter

1 ½ cups distilled water

Instructions:

Put all ingredients in a blender. Whiz on high speed until smooth. Pour into glasses and serve immediately.

Variation: Substitute pitted dates with 1 tablespoon of raw coconut nectar or raw agave nectar Add 1 cup of ice cubes for a cold treat.

Mint not only triggers a feeling of satiety (it makes you feel full!) but also helps flush out toxins from the digestive tract. It also aids in proper digestion by soothing the intestines and loosening intestinal muscles, thus relieving cramps and other symptoms of disturbed stomach.

Tropical Blast Green Smoothie

Ingredients:

1 cup of pineapple

1 cup of mango

1 cup of banana

¾ cup of spinach

2 cups of fresh coconut water, almond milk, or clean, filtered water

6 ice cubes (optional)

Instructions:

Make sure to thoroughly rinse and clean the spinach in clean water. Dice the pineapple, mango and banana to measure one cup. Add all ingredients to your blender (add spinach last). Blend for 30 seconds to 1 minute, depending on speed setting. Let the ingredients blend until creamy.

Mangoes are highly effective in soothing the GI tract and optimizing your digestion. Furthermore, the pretty fruits are rich in vitamin C, providing an essential immune system boost. Pineapples contribute to weight loss because they have a very high water and fiber content. High water/fiber content foods make you feel satisfied; so another snack is not necessary. Furthermore, pineapples have been shown to naturally curb your appetite.

Savory & Spicy Green Smoothie

Ingredients:

1 whole avocado

1 lemon

1 orange beet (small)

1 cucumber (small)

5 stalks of collards greens

2 drops of vanilla extract

1 inch-thick piece of ginger

½ of a jalapeno pepper

Instructions:

Remove the seeds and skin from the lemon, and add them to the blender. Cut cucumber, orange beet, and collard greens into smaller chunks, then add the collard greens to the blender last. Place the ginger, avocado, jalapeno (with seeds) and clean water in the blender's pitcher last. Blend until the green smoothie reaches your desired consistency. *Wash the collards, cucumber, and jalapeno thoroughly before adding to blender.

Jalapeno peppers lend an essential nutritional punch to your green smoothie. One of the jalapeno pepper's key nutrients is capsaicin; it revs your metabolism and boosts your immune system. It further increases your blood flow, weight loss capabilities, and boosts your energy. Ginger is excellent to ward off cancers and interior muscle soreness. It further works to alleviate nausea. This smoothie also serves as a great meal replacement for breakfast; it's rich and filling and will keep you full and energized throughout a busy morning. It will also decrease your likelihood of snacking on other processed foods!

Coconut Pumpkin Green Smoothie

Ingredients:

2/3 cup of pumpkin puree

1 1/2 tbsp. coconut oil

1 cup almond milk, or coconut water (or clean water)

1 medium-sized pear

1 cup spinach

1 tbsp. Avocado (optional)

1 cup red seedless grapes

Instructions:

First thoroughly wash spinach, grapes, and the pear in water with a bit of vinegar (vinegar helps to clean more impurities from the produce). Add the tbsp. of avocado, grapes, pear, almond milk (or coconut water), coconut oil, water, and then blend. While blending, slowly add the pumpkin puree and then the lettuce. Allow it to blend until smooth and creamy.

Pumpkin puree is that delicious secret-ingredient, bringing pumpkin pie flavor to your next green smoothie. With this serving-size of pumpkin puree, you will be getting about 6 times the daily recommended amount of Vitamin A, essential for eye, lung, heart, and kidney health. Coconut oil is also great for facilitating weight loss. It's rich in medium chain triglycerides (MCFAs), which increase the liver's rate of metabolism by up to 30 percent, according to various research studies.

Strawberry-Coconut Green Smoothie

Ingredients:

1 cup of strawberries (fresh or frozen)

1/2 lemon (without skin)

2 kale leaves (without stem)

1 cup of coconut water

1.5 tbsp. coconut oil

1 tbsp. hemp seeds

Instructions:

First allow the strawberries (if using fresh) and kale to soak in a bowl of water with a dash of vinegar (for better cleaning). Then add the coconut oil, coconut water, hemp seeds, lemon, and strawberries to the blender. After chopping the kale into smaller pieces, add it last. Blend until your desired consistency.

Omega-3 fatty acids are critical for the overall health and functionality of our brain, bodily cells, and hormones. In order to ensure long-term health, you should make it a goal to consume either hemp or Chia seeds every day. Lemons are amazing liver detoxifiers; fueling the liver with greater health is essential in order to digest and burn fat. Furthermore, despite their acidic taste, they act to alkalize bodily fluids and tissues.

"Kickstart" Green Smoothie

Ingredients:

1 cup of fresh pineapple

1 lime (peeled, seeds removed)

2 inch-thick piece of ginger root

½ bunch of parsley

1 cup of romaine lettuce

½ medium-sized cucumber

1 cup of filtered water or coconut water

Instructions:

After thoroughly rinsing the parsley, romaine and cucumber, add them to the blender except the romaine. Also add the ginger, coconut water, pineapple, lime, and the lettuce last. Blend until it reaches your desired consistency.

The three key ingredients in this digestion kick-starter smoothie are pineapple, ginger, and lime. Pineapple boasts a certain enzyme otherwise known as bromelain, which is beneficial for enhancing the digestive flow. Ginger is particularly good for promoting the production of good bacteria in the GI tract; it further works to get rid of bad bacteria that causes constipation. Lime is a great overall detoxifier that helps to eliminate unwanted pathogens and parasites from the colon.

Mango-Lemon Delight Green Smoothie

Ingredients:

1 cup of fresh mango

2 cups of kale

1 lime (peeled, seeds removed)

⅓ bunch of cilantro

1 tbsp. of hemp seeds

1 cup of filtered water

Instructions:

After adding some water and a bit of vinegar (for enhanced cleaning effects) to a large mixing bowl, allow the lettuce and cilantro to rinse until they are without impurities. Then in the blender, add the water, lime, hemp seeds, mango, cilantro and lettuce (make sure the lettuce is added last) and blend until the smoothie is mixed to your desired consistency.

Mangoes provide essential digestive assistance. They have a wide array of enzymes that are good for soothing the digestive walls and releasing toxic build-up. Furthermore, they are abundant in vitamins such as A and C, which can help to protect the body from free-radical damage and premature aging.

Citrus Punch Detox Smoothie

Ingredients:
2 kale leaves (without stems)
½ cup of chopped cilantro
1 lime (peeled, seeds removed)
1 large-sized banana
½ red grapefruit
2 small oranges
1 lemon (peeled, seeds removed)
1 to 2 cups of filtered water (depending on your desired consistency.)

Instructions:
Thoroughly wash the cilantro and kale before preparing it for your blender. Peel the skin and deseed the lemon, lime, oranges and grapefruit, and then add them to the blender. Add the banana. Thoroughly wash the cilantro and kale leaves, and then place them in the blender along with the clean water. Blend until you reach desired consistency.

Citrus fruits detox your body of unwanted mucus. When your body relieves itself of unwanted mucus, it will have the ability to fuel itself with proper nutrients from the foods you eat. Too much mucus in the body disallows this ready nutrient absorption.

Electrolyte Balancer Green Smoothie

Ingredients:

2 cups of fresh pineapple

2 fresh celery ribs, chopped

1 cup of spinach

1 lime (without skin and seeds)

2 cups of coconut milk

Instructions:

Before adding the celery and spinach to the blender, first thoroughly soak & rinse them with water. Then in the blender's pitcher, add the chopped pineapple chunks, celery, lime, coconut milk and spinach; allow all of the fresh ingredients to blend until they reach a creamy, smooth texture.

When you want to enhance your electrolyte and hormonal balance, you must look to the beneficial effects of both coconut milk and celery. Furthermore, when you add pineapple, this smoothie fights back against certain strains of bacteria and infections. It further acts as nourishment for both your hair and skin.

Orange-Banana Green Smoothie

Ingredients:

1 cup spinach

1 large banana

2 celery ribs

2 oranges (peeled)

1 coconut water or filtered water

Instructions:

Allow the spinach and celery to soak in water to remove any impurities. Afterwards, add oranges, celery, banana, and coconut water to the blender. Make sure to add the spinach last, and allow the mix to blend until it is creamy enough for your preference.

If you're opting for orange's pulsing nutrients, it's best to look to the natural variety for assistance. Store-bought orange juice has been sitting on the shelves for days and days. Many orange juice products consist of only water and synthetic orange flavoring (with no nutrition at all!). When you utilize freshly blended or juiced oranges, you are getting a higher value of vitamin A & C, both of which are crucial for your body to fend off toxins, pathogens, and bacteria. Remember: when it comes to fruits and vegetables, fresh is always best!

Sweet Kiwi Green Smoothie

Ingredients:

2 leaves kale (without stems)

1 medium cucumber (peeled)

2 kiwis (without skin)

2 Medjool dates (pitted)

1 cup of coconut water (or clean water)

Instructions:

First wash the kale and cucumber. Dice both and add the cucumber to the blender, along with the kiwis, dates and coconut water. Add the kale last while blending. Allow the mixture of fruits and vegetables to blend until they reach your desired consistency.

The vibrant green kiwis contain high levels of omega 3 fatty acids, something usually found in nuts and very rarely in fruits. Remember that your brain requires a balance in the brain of omega-3 fatty acids because they create better cell-to-cell communication, fueling necessary hormonal balances. Furthermore, kiwis are a great source of potassium and vitamin C. Recent research states that kiwis are especially effective in the prevention of cellular oxidation. Remember that cellular oxidation is the event in which free radicals kill cells by removing one of their electrons and forcing protein and DNA death. This hinders the cell's ability to communicate with surrounding cells and eventually kills it. Cucumbers contain silica, a trace mineral that increases the body's ability to heal skin wounds. This mineral can also assist with strengthening the skin's connective tissues.

Hemp Protein Cinnamon Green Smoothie

Ingredients:

½ cup blueberries

¼ cup strawberries

¼ cup coconut milk

1 cup de-stalked kale

1 tbsp. hemp protein powder

1 tbsp. flax seed

2 tbsp. chia seeds

1 ½ tsp. cinnamon

1 ½ tbsp. acai

1 banana

Instructions:

Begin by placing the blueberries, strawberries, and peeled banana together in the blender. Blend for five seconds. Next, add in the coconut milk, the flax seed, the chia seeds, cinnamon, hemp protein powder, and the acai. Blend for ten seconds. Add the kale at the very end, and blend the mixture until it reaches your desired consistency. Enjoy this nutritive, green protein smoothie.

This smoothie yields the essential benefits of the superfood, hemp, via the hemp protein powder. Furthermore, this smoothie purports another superfood, acai, a berry that contains all the nutritive goodness of the marriage between fruit and chocolate. It further boasts essential fatty acids that fuel greater brain communication. Look to the delicious recipe below for weight loss and a ready boost of brain activity.

Chia Kiwi Green Power Smoothie

Ingredients:

1 cup almond milk

1 banana

1 ¾ cups spinach

1 diced kiwi

1 tbsp. chia seeds

1 tsp. maca powder

2 ½ tbsp. wheatgrass powder

Instructions:

Begin by bringing the almond milk, spinach, banana, and the diced kiwi together in a blender. Next, add the chia seeds, maca powder, and the wheatgrass powder for extra pizzaz. Blend until you achieve desired consistency.

This chia kiwi green power smoothie is rushing with iron-heavy spinach, good fats from almond milk, awesome phytonutrients from the chia seeds, and wheatgrass, a superfood that yields tons of vitamin C, vitamin A, calcium, magnesium, potassium, and phosphorus. Just like spinach and kale, it is rich with chlorophyll, which brings remarkable detox and weight loss benefits to your body.

Citrus Kale Protein Smoothie

Ingredients:
¼ cup red grapefruit juice
1 diced apple
1 ½ cups de-stemmed kale
1 diced celery stalk
1 cup diced cucumber
½ cup mango
4 tbsp. hemp hearts
¼ cup mint leaves
4 ice cubes
½ tbsp. coconut oil

Instructions:
Begin by juicing the grapefruit and adding its juice to the blender. Next, toss in the cucumber, kale, apple, hemp hearts, celery, mango, mint, coconut oil, and the ice. Blend the ingredients until they reach your desired consistency. Enjoy immediately.

Hemp hearts, a formulation of our old superfood, hemp seeds, appear in this protein smoothie, yielding the ideal omega-3 and omega-6 fatty acid balance your brain requires for ready communication and hormone health. Furthermore, hemp hearts are high in fiber. The incredible balance between apples, mangoes, and grapefruit alongside the non-obtrusive taste of the kale is undeniably brilliant.

Green Vegie Drink

Ingredients:

2 cups spinach

1/2 cucumber

1/4 head of celery

1/2 bunch parsley

1 bunch mint

3 carrots

Instructions:

1. Combine all ingredients in a blender.
2. Add water to get desired consistency and drink fresh.

Spinach contains an antioxidant known as alpha-lipoic acid, which lower glucose levels, increase insulin sensitivity and prevent oxidative stress-induced changes in patients with diabetes and decreases peripheral neuropathy in diabetics.

Mango Smoothie

Ingredients:

¼ c. mango cubes

¼ c. mashed ripe avocado

½ c. mango juice

¼ c. fat-free vanilla yogurt

1 tbsp. freshly squeezed lime juice

Instructions:

1. Combine all ingredients in a blender and process until smooth.
2. Pour into a tall glass.
3. Garnish with sliced mango or strawberry.
4. Drink fresh

Mango prevents cancer, lowers cholesterol, improves eye health, alkalizes the body, may help with diabetes, may help to promote healthy sex drive, improves digestion, helps fight heat stroke, boosts the immune system.

Slimming Green Smoothie

Ingredients:

6 fl. Oz. Unsweetened almond milk

1/3 banana

1/2 cup pineapple, fresh or frozen

1 tbsp. almond or peanut butter

Instructions:

1. Add ingredients to Four Side or Wild Side + jar in order listed and secure lid.

2. Select "Smoothie".

3. Drink fresh.

Bananas help overcome depression, sustain blood sugar, gives energy, protect against muscle cramps, build strong bones due to their calcium content, reduce swelling, help strengthen the nervous system, contain high levels of vitamin B-6, potassium, low in salt, protect against heart attack and stroke.

Blueberry Smoothie

Ingredients:

1 c skim milk

1 c frozen unsweetened blueberries

Instructions:

1. Combine milk and blueberries in blender, and blend for 1 minute.
2. Transfer to glass, and stir in flaxseed oil.
3. Drink fresh.

Blueberries considered a "superfood", are low in calories but high in nutrients and super healthy. They contain Fiber, Vitamin C, Vitamin K and Manganese. Blueberries reduce DNA damage, which may help protect against ageing and cancer, lower blood pressure, protect LDL lipoproteins (the "bad" cholesterol) from oxidative damage, prevent heart disease, improve brain function and memory, has anti-diabetic effects, prevents urinary tract infections, help reduce muscle damage after intensive exercise.

Apple Low Carb Smoothie

Ingredients:

2 large green apples cored

1 frozen banana

1 cup ice

1 cup unsweetened almond milk

1/ 2 cup Greek yogurt

Instructions:

1. Add all ingredients to a blender.
2. Pulse until combined and smooth.
3. Taste and add sweetener if desired, pulsing to combine.
4. Serve immediately.
5. Sprinkle the top of each smoothie with a pinch of cinnamon.
6. Drink fresh.

"An apple a day keeps the doctor away". Apples are known to improve neurological health, prevent dementia, reduce the risk of stroke, reduce the risk of diabetes, help prevent breast cancer, prevent bad cholesterol in blood from rising, protect the body from the free radicals.

Detox Green Smoothie

Ingredients:

1 stalk kale, stem removed

1 cup baby spinach/ greens

1/ 2 lemon, seeds removed, skin on

1/ 2 inch piece of peeled ginger

3 inch piece of peeled cucumber

Instructions:

1. Combine all ingredients in a blender and blend until smooth.

2. Drink fresh.

Kale is high in iron, in Vitamin K, filled with powerful antioxidants, has anti-inflammatory properties and cardiovascular support substances, high in Vitamin A, Vitamin C, calcium and is a great detox food, keeping the liver healthy.

Pineapple Spinach Detox Smoothie

Ingredients:

3/ 4 cup pineapple juice

1/ 2 cup fresh spinach leaves

1/ 4 pear, chopped

1/ 4 green apple, chopped

1/ 4 avocado, chopped

Instructions:

1. Blend pineapple juice, spinach, pear, apple, avocado, and broccoli together in a blender until smooth.
2. Drink fresh.

Pineapples improves respiratory health, improves digestion, strengthens bones, reduces inflammation, prevents cancer, increases heart health, reduces infections and parasites, strengthens the immune system, and increases circulation.

Pear Avocado Smoothie

Ingredients:
½ pear
¼ avocado
½ cucumber
½ lemon
handful of cilantro
1 cup kale (packed)
½ inch ginger
½ cup coconut water
1 scoop protein powder (hemp, pumpkin or pea works great!)
Water

Instructions:
1. Blend all ingredients until smooth.
2. Drink fresh.

The health benefits of avocado include weight management, protection against cardiovascular diseases, diabetes, osteoarthritis and enhancing the absorption of nutrients. It also reduces the risk of cancer, liver damage and Vitamin K deficiency-related bleeding. Keeps eyes healthy and protects the skin from aging and from harmful effects of UV rays. It also helps in maintaining normal blood sugar levels and has antioxidant properties, boosts cognitive abilities, and build stronger bones!

Papaya Smoothie

Ingredients:

1 cup papaya

1 cup coconut kefir, coconut yogurt or coconut milk

juice from ½ lime

1 tbsp. raw honey

Instructions:

1. Blend all ingredients until smooth.
2. Drink fresh.

Papaya is rich in fiber, improves digestion, rich in Vitamin C and antioxidants, lowers cholesterol, boosts immunity, good for diabetics, great for the eyes, protects against arthritis, prevents signs of ageing and cancer and helps reduce stress.

Pear Avocado Smoothie with Chia Seeds

Ingredients:

½ pear

¼ avocado

1 packed cup spinach

¼ cup coconut water

1 cup almond milk

1 tsp chia seeds

1 scoop protein powder

Water

Instructions:

1. Blend all ingredients together until smooth.

2. Drink fresh.

Chia seeds excel in their high amount of antioxidants, almost all the carbs in them are fiber. Chia Seeds are high in protein, Omega-3 Fatty Acids and they lower the risk of heart disease and Type 2 Diabetes. They are high in calcium, phosphorus, magnesium and protein.

Apple Avocado Smoothie with Hemp Seeds

Ingredients:

1 apple, cored

1/ 4 avocado, peeled

2 tablespoons hemp seeds

2 cups baby spinach

8 ounces (236 ml) unsweetened almond milk

Instructions:

1. Combine the ingredients into a good powerful blender until smooth and creamy.

2. Drink fresh.

Hemp seeds are good for heart and mind and are also a rich source of a number of essential minerals, including magnesium, phosphorus, iron and zinc, full of fiber that improves bowel function by helping prevent constipation. Hemp seeds contain 20 amino acids, including the 9 essential amino acids (EAAs) our bodies cannot produce.

Cholesterol Reducing Green Smoothie

Ingredients:

2 cups spinach or kale

1 apple

½ avocado cut in half

Spoon half into blender

1 tsp Spirulina powder

Instructions:

1. Chuck the ingredients into your blender keeping the same order.

2. Blend for at least 1 min until smooth.

3. Drink fresh.

Spirulina is actually bacteria, or blue - green algae that are found in freshwater lakes, ponds, and rivers. Spirulina strengthen the immune system, is exceptionally important for healthy eyes, helps improve the Digestive System. It has been shown to be effective at helping remove toxins from the blood, and it binds to heavy metals and radioactive.

Green Smoothie with Spinach, Mango and Mint

Ingredients:

1 good handful of fresh spinach

2 ripe mangos

3-4 twigs of fresh mint

2 lime fruits

Ice

Water

Instructions:

1. Put the peeled and roughly chopped fruit and herbs in the blender along with some ice and water

2. Blend until smooth

3. Cool and serve.

Mint is a great appetizer, promotes digestion and activates the salivary glands. Mint can be very soothing for nausea and related motion sickness. Use of mint is very beneficial for asthma, depression and fatigue, improves levels of memory and may help prevent and treat cancer.

Green Juicy Smoothie

Ingredients:

A bunch of fresh spinach

3 sticks of celery

3 apples

1 pear

1 lemon

Instructions:

1. Put it all through the blender.
2. Add some water and blend until smooth.
3. Drink fresh.

Pears are among the less allergenic of all the fruits, and able to lower blood pressure and cholesterol levels. Traditional medicines use them in the treatment of colitis, chronic gallbladder disorders, arthritis, and gout. They help with weight loss and reduce the risk of developing cancer, hypertension, diabetes, heart disease, coronary disease and type 2 diabetes.

Shiro Plum & Kale Energizer

Ingredients:

2 cups kale

2 shiro plums

1/ 2 cup fresh raspberries or strawberries

1/ 4 cup oats

1 teaspoon flax seed

¼ cup raisins

¼ cup nuts

½ cup water

1 cup ice.

Instructions: Blend the kale together with the plums, oats, raisins, nuts and water for around 2 minutes before adding the raspberries. After half a minute of mixing just add the rest of the ingredients and blend until smooth.

Ingredients:

1 cup spinach

1 banana

1/ 2 cup coconut milk

1 teaspoon walnut oil

1 teaspoon flax seed

1 tablespoon dry coconut

1 cup of ice.

Instructions: It's probably best to blend the banana and spinach first before adding the coconut milk together with the rest of the ingredients. You can add ½ a cup of fresh pineapple in the mix as it's always a good combination with banana and coconut.

Seriously Cool Slushy

Ingredients:

250ml baby kale leaves

½ cup homemade, unsweetened applesauce or pear sauce

500ml water or coconut water

250ml organic lemonade

This is awesome on a hot summer's day. It has a fair amount of sugar in it so it should also be kept as an occasional treat. What I sometimes do is to freeze this mixture to make lollipops for the kiddies.

Apple Greens Smoothie

Ingredients:

1 cup red apple, cored & sliced with skin on

½ celery stalk coarsely chopped

½ cup kale coarsely chopped

½ cup cilantro coarsely chopped

tbsp. fresh lemon juice

½ tsp. ground ginger

1 cup apple juice

Instructions:

Blend the leafy greens and liquids first at low speed for 1 minute. Add the fruits and harder chunks. Blend at slow speed for 1 minute. Move to medium speed continue blending for 1 minute. Blend at high speed for 1 minute.

Apple Pear & Kiwi Smoothie

Ingredients:

1 cups apple with skin on chopped

2 cups pear chopped

½ cup kiwi

½ cup ice cubes

1/ 4 cup water

1 (1 inch) piece peeled fresh ginger

¼ cups fresh mint leaves coarsely chopped

Instructions:

Blend leafy greens and liquids at low speed for 1 minute. Add the fruits and all other ingredients to the blender. Blend at slow speed for 1 minute. Move to medium speed until and continue blending for 1 minute. Finish blending at high speed for another minute.

Apple Celery & Cilantro Smoothie

Ingredients:

1 cup apples coarsely chopped with skin on

½ cup celery coarsely chopped

¼ cup cilantro pinch of c cinnamon

½ tsp. ground ginger juice of ½ lime

1 cup water

Instructions:

Blend leafy greens and liquids at low speed for 1 minute. Add the fruits and all other ingredients to the blender. Blend at slow speed for 1 minute. Move to medium speed until and continue blending for 1 minute. Finish blending at high speed for another minute.

The Hempy

Ingredients:
2 tbsp hemp protein powder
¾ cup spinach, chopped
¾ cup fresh mango, cubed
½ cup strawberries, sliced
1 large celery stalk, chopped
½ cup tangerine
¼ cup parsley, chopped
Ice (optional)

Instructions:
1. Add all of the ingredients to the blender, and puree until all of the ingredients become completely smooth.
2. Pour into your favorite glass and enjoy!

Your digestive system will thank you for this smoothie! The sweetness of the mango, strawberries, and tangerine together makes it hard to believe that this is a Super Green Smoothie. Hemp is a highly recommended vegetable protein that contains HIGH QUALITY dietary plant protein. Dietary protein is essential your body's healthy growth and maintenance.

Kiwi Detox Smoothie

Ingredients:

4 kiwi, peeled and quartered

2 tbsp hemp protein

½ cup hemp yogurt

1 cup Good Karma Flax Milk

½ Cup Blueberries

2 Ice Cubes

Instructions:

1. Add all of the ingredients to the blender, and puree until all of the ingredients become completely smooth.

2. Pour into your favorite glass and enjoy!

This is a nutrient dense smoothie that will give you the energy you need to make it through the morning rush. It just so happens to be graced with the presence of kiwi, which is rich in disease fighting anti-oxidants. Kiwis have a special super power that allows them to bind and move those nasty toxins in your digestive tract out of the way. If consumed on a frequent basis will make constipation a thing of the past.

Sweet Green Smoothie

Ingredients:

2 c coconut water, frozen into cubes

¼ c lime juice

½ Hass avocado

¼ c shredded coconut, unsweetened

1 c fresh spinach, tightly packed

1 tbsp agave OR honey (OR 1 tsp liquid sweetener of your choice)

3 dates, pitted

Instructions:

Add all ingredients to your blender, frozen coconut water should be split between top and bottom of blender canister. Blend on low, slowly building up to high. Blend until smooth and creamy.

Spinach for fiber and iron, coconut and avocado for good fats and energy as well as coconut and dates for sweetness? Who could ask for more in this nutrition packed punch of flavor brought together by the tantalizing tang of lime.

Favorite Spinach Green Smoothie

Ingredients:

1 banana, peeled, frozen and sliced

½ c your choice of frozen berries

1 tbsp flaxseed meal

1-2 tbsp peanut butter

¾ c unsweetened almond milk, vanilla flavored

2 c fresh spinach

Instructions:

Blend all ingredients together until creamy. You can add more milk if you want it thinner or bananas if you prefer your smoothie thicker. Drink it immediately or freeze it to enjoy later.

Get ready to have your mind blown. This green smoothie doesn't taste anything like spinach so it makes a wonderfully healthy breakfast. Sweet, creamy and extremely satisfying, it will give you the energy you need to get through your busy morning.

Classic Green Smoothie

Ingredients:

1 c almond milk

2 c fresh spinach, tightly packed

2 bananas, sliced and frozen

2 tbsp ground flax seed

1 tbsp chia seeds

3 ice cubes

Instructions:

Toss all the ingredients in the blender in the order listed. Blend until smooth.

This smoothie offers nearly half of your daily recommended amount of calcium. It is also one of the most filling and satisfying smoothies to drink for when you just don't have time to fit a meal into your hectic schedule.

Green Warrior Protein Smoothie

Ingredients:

½ c orange juice

1 c kale, tightly packed

1 lg apple, chopped; your choice of Fuji, Gala or Jonathan

1 c cucumber, chopped

½ c celery, chopped

3 tbsp ground hemp seeds

1 tbsp chia seeds

1 mango, cubed and frozen

3 tbsp fresh mint leaves

1 tbsp coconut butter

4 ice cubes

Instructions:

Place all ingredients as listed in your blender. Blend until smooth. Scrape the sides of the canister as necessary. If this smoothie is too thick you can add more orange juice or a little coconut water to thin it down.

Are you having trouble getting all those leafy green vegetables you need? This smoothie is just packed with the vitamins and minerals from the combination of kale, cucumbers, apples and so much more. It's perfect for drinking just before your strength training or for being able to stick to your diet.

Green Apple Pie Smoothie

Ingredients:

1 c apple cider

1 tbsp walnuts, ground

½ tsp cinnamon

¼ tsp vanilla or maple extract

1/8 tsp nutmeg

2 c spinach, tightly packed

2 lg apples, chopped and frozen; your choice of Jonathan, Fuji or Gala

½ Hass avocado, peeled, chopped and frozen

Instructions:

Blend all ingredients together until smooth. If it is still too thin you can add 4-6 ice cubes or 1 scoop of vanilla flavored protein powder.

Do you love apple pie but hate what it does to your waistline? Well this apple pie smoothie is simple to make, creamy, sweet and absolutely indulgent. The best part is – it's low in calories!

Green Tea Power Smoothie

Ingredients:

1 cucumber, seeded, sliced and frozen

3 c fresh spinach, tightly packed

2 c honeydew melon, cubed and frozen (about ½ a melon)

1 c brewed green tea

1 tsp lemon juice

½ inch fresh ginger root, peeled and minced

Instructions:

Blend all ingredients together and enjoy! You can freeze the green tea into cubes if you want a thicker smoothie. For a creamier drink, add 1 c coconut milk. For additional energy and more protein than the spinach provides, add 2 scoops vanilla flavored protein powder.

Brew a pot of green tea and have it in the refrigerator for when you need a quick energy boost or a sweet and easy breakfast when you're on the go. Juicy melon, refreshing cucumber, energizing spinach and warming ginger root all combine to make this one of the best smoothies you'll ever taste.

Green-Power Smoothie

Ingredients:

1 c green tea, brewed and cooled

1 c honeydew melon, cubed and frozen

1 plum, pitted

20 green grapes, peeled and frozen (for sweetness)

½ cucumber, peeled, seeded and cubed

½ c fresh spinach, tightly packed

2 tbsp chia seeds

4 ice cubes

Instructions:

Place all ingredients into the canister of your blender. Pulse to break up larger pieces and then puree until smooth.

You'll be amazed at how this smoothie makes you feel. Tons of green power and less than 200 calories! Have your green tea brewed and refrigerated and you'll be ready to hit the door running in no time.

Ultra Green Smoothie

Ingredients:

1 c plain yogurt

2 c fresh spinach, tightly packed

½ Hass avocado, cubed and frozen

1 banana, sliced and frozen

2 tbsp hemp seeds

3 ice cubes

Instructions:

Blend all ingredients until smooth. Serve and enjoy!

Are you tired of plateauing on your weight loss plan? This smoothie is packed with nutrition that will get your guts moving in the right direction which will help you get back on track.

Tropical Green Smoothie

Ingredients:

2 c coconut water

1 mango, peeled, pitted, cubed and frozen

1 c pineapple chunks, frozen

2 c fresh spinach, tightly packed

¼ c fresh mint leaves, tightly packed and stems removed

1 tbsp lime juice

10 ice cubes

Instructions:

Add all ingredients to your blender, beginning on low speed work up to high until smooth.

This sweet-tart smoothie comes with a tropical twist that will have you doing the limbo in no time. Sweet mango and tangy pineapple mingle with mint and lime that will make you forget this smoothie is healthy!

Kale Strawberry Kiwi

You can sub nearly any green for the dandelion.

Ingredients:

1 cup fresh kale greens

1 cup fresh dandelion greens

2 cups fresh orange juice

2 cups strawberries

2 kiwis (peeled or unpeeled)

1 banana

1 squeezed lemon

Instructions:

Thoroughly wash the applicable fruits and vegetables. Blend the kale, dandelion and orange juice until smooth. Add the other ingredients and blend until smooth. You can optionally add ice or freeze one of the ingredients to make the drink cold. Serve.

Minty Avocado Smoothie

Ingredients:

1 small avocado, peeled and pitted

4 mint leaves

1 cup coconut milk

1 tablespoon erythritol

1 tablespoon colostrum powder

Instructions:

Combine all the ingredients in a blender and pulse until smooth and creamy. Serve the smoothie as fresh as possible.

This refreshing smoothie is amazing for your morning meals. Thick and creamy, it will keep you full for a longer time, while the mint will awaken your senses and force them to work at their highest peaks.

Lemon Green Tea Smoothie

Ingredients:

2 tablespoons lemon juice

1 tablespoon organic Matcha powder

1 cup coconut water

1/2 cup coconut milk

1 tablespoon erythritol

1 tablespoon MCT oil

Instructions:

Mix all the ingredients in a blender and pulse until smooth. Pour the drink in glasses and serve it as fresh as possible.

Green tea is an excellent source of antioxidants and including it into your diet is a great idea, especially in the morning when your body needs a restart and enough nutrients to feed on for the rest of the day. Use green tea powder – Match – for a quicker smoothie.

Celery Cauliflower Smoothie

Ingredients:

2 celery stalks

1 cup cauliflower florets

1 cup coconut milk

1 tablespoon raw almonds

4 ice cubes

Instructions:

Mix all the ingredients in a blender until smooth and creamy. Pour the drink in glasses and serve it as fresh as possible.

This savory smoothie is thick and refreshing and to be honest, it could easily count as a dish on its own if topped with even more vegetables, such as avocado or cilantro.

Lemon Cucumber Smoothie

Ingredients:

1 large cucumber

1 lemon, juiced

1/2 teaspoon lemon zest

1 cup coconut water

1 tablespoon erythritol

1 tablespoon MCT oil

Instructions:

Mix all the ingredients in a blender and pulse until smooth.
Pour the drink in glasses and serve it as fresh as possible.

This watery, refreshing smoothie will re-balance your system
and boost your energy right away. Remember that keeping
your body hydrated is crucial during this diet and any other diet
for that matter.

Cilantro Limeade Smoothie

Ingredients:

1 cup fresh cilantro

1 lemon, juiced

1/2 teaspoon grated ginger

1 1/2 cups coconut water

1/4 cup cashew nuts, soaked overnight

Instructions:

Mix all the ingredients in a powerful blender. Pulse until smooth and creamy. Pour the drink in glasses and serve it as fresh as possible.

This light and refreshing smoothie will surely awake your senses in the morning. In addition to that, it is great for metabolism and loaded with antioxidants.

Avocado and Broccoli Smoothie

Ingredients:

1 cup watercress

1 cup cubed beetroot

1 cup broccoli florets, blanched

1 avocado, pitted and peeled

1/ 2 Tbsp. hulled sesame seeds

1 cup unsweetened almond milk

Instructions: Place the sesame seeds in the Nutribullet and blend until ground. Add the watercress, beetroot, broccoli, avocado, and almond milk. Blend until

Super Green Smoothie

Ingredients:
2 cups baby spinach
1 cucumber, sliced
1 avocado, peeled and pitted
1 celery stalk
1/4 cup cilantro
1 lemon, juiced
1 cup coconut water

Instructions:
Soften the spinach in a steamer for 5 minutes then transfer it in a blender. Add the cucumber, avocado, celery, cilantro, lemon juice and water in a blender. Pulse until smooth and creamy and pour the drink in glasses and serve it as fresh as possible.

Since raw spinach is not allowed in some diets, here is a small trick: softened spinach in a steamer for a few minutes before blending it into the smoothie.

Hydrating Celery Smoothie

Ingredients:

2 celery stalks, chopped

1 cucumber, sliced

1 1/2 cups coconut water

2 mint leaves

4 ice cubes

1 tablespoon MCT oil

Instructions:

Mix all the ingredients in a blender. Pulse until smooth and creamy and serve the smoothie as fresh as possible.

Liquids are extremely important for any diet, not just this particular one, but apart from water, you can also come up with this kind of drinks that are hydrating and nutritious at the same time.

Prunes and Greens Smoothie

Ingredients:

1 cup prunes, stoned

1 cup spinach

1 cup sliced green beans, blanched

1 cup broccoli florets, blanched

1 Tbsp. walnuts

1 cup unsweetened almond milk

Instructions:

Place the walnuts in the Nutribullet and blend until ground. Add the prunes, spinach, green beans, broccoli, and almond milk. Blend until you get a smooth

Ingredients:

1 cup unsweetened almond milk

1/ 2 cup frozen pineapple

2 cups kale

1/ 2 banana

1 cup frozen peaches

Instructions:

Prepare all the ingredients and put them in a blender. Pulse on medium speed. Process until smooth. When the mixture becomes smooth and creamy, transfer it into your glass and serve.

Power up your day with powerful combinations of fruits such as peaches, pineapples, bananas, and spinach. Peaches is a good source of antioxidants with a long list of benefits including its anti-inflammatory, anti-cancer, and anti-aging effects. Banana, on the other hand, is rich in potassium. You also have pineapples with bromelain, which aids in inflammation and is good for the heart. Top all these with spinach and you are in for some flavorful and nutritious smoothie.

Kiwi and Guava Smoothie

Ingredients:

1 kiwi fruit, sliced

1 guava, sliced

2 /3 cup coconut water

¼ cup crushed ice

Instructions:

Prepare all the ingredients and put them in a blender. Pulse on medium speed. Process until smooth. When the mixture becomes smooth and creamy, transfer it into your glass and serve.

If you want to have an improved immune system, you have to try the powerful combinations of guava and kiwi smoothie. This drink is rich in phytonutrients that helps fight against cancer cells. Kiwi is chockfull of vitamins and minerals that helps against cancer formation. Guava, on the other hand, helps strengthens the immune system and protects the body against free radicals. Combine it with coconut to give the smoothie a rich and creamy texture. Try this recipe and experience its goodness.

Green Tea Smoothie with Cucumber and Kale

Ingredients:

1 cup green tea, chilled

1 cup cucumber

1 cup loosely packed cilantro

1 cup pineapple

1 tablespoon ginger, grated

1 cup baby kale

juice of 1 lemon

½ avocado

Instructions:

Prepare all the ingredients and put them in a blender. Pulse on medium speed. Process until smooth. When the mixture becomes smooth and creamy, transfer it into your glass and serve.

Orange and Kale Green Smoothie

Ingredients:

1 cup chopped raw kale

1 orange, peeled and deseeded

1 pinch of ground cinnamon

1 pinch of ginger powder

1 cup water

Instructions:

Prepare all the ingredients and put them in a blender. Pulse on medium speed.Process until smooth. When the mixture becomes smooth and creamy, transfer it into your glass and serve.

This smoothie acts two ways – energizes and detoxifies your body. This is perfect for those who are looking for a detox drink.